Common Thyroid Disease Complications

Secondary Problems Needing Special Attention

By: James M. Lowrance © 2010

INTRODUCTION:

There are basically two categories of thyroid dysfunction, the one being an under-active thyroid gland or "hypothyroidism" and the other being an overactive thyroid gland or "hyperthyroidism".

Both conditions of thyroid hormone imbalance can develop due to a number of different causes and both have treatments that can return the abnormally high or abnormally low levels of thyroid hormones, back-to the normal values range (optimally when possible).

The goal of these treatments is to restore a patient's bodily metabolism, so that it functions at the best possible level.

While a patient may see their thyroid dysfunction resolved over time, they may potentially experience secondary complications of their thyroid diseases that will require special attention and/or additional treatments.

In this book, I will be addressing a number of these type issues, many being common thyroid disease complications with others being less common or rare.

It is important that thyroid patients be made aware of both the common and rare types of complications because some of these have better treatment outcomes, the earlier they can be diagnosed and treated.

TABLE OF CONTENTS:

CHAPTER ONE

Hair Loss

A symptom that is listed for both hypothyroid and hyperthyroid conditions is "hair loss". Some patients, especially those with hyperthyroidism, may see rapid hair loss with their thyroid disorder. Other patients only see mild to moderate hair loss, such as finding more hair in the sink after washing it. Hypothyroid patients will find that their hair becomes dry and brittle and will also break off rather than just falling out.

Some thyroid patients being treated for hypothyroidism will report that they experience hair loss, more so with a particular type of thyroid hormone replacement medication.

The hair loss they experienced prior to starting hormone therapy was mild to moderate or in some cases almost unnoticeable but once starting thyroid medication, they see a rapid increase in hair loss.

I have seen this attested to, more often in patients taking synthetic forms of thyroid hormone medications.

Other patients are not affected in regard to hair loss by synthetic or the natural types (animal derived) of thyroid hormone medications.

In my case, as a hypothyroid patient, I experienced mild hair loss when I began to experience symptoms of hypothyroidism from Hashimoto's thyroiditis (autoimmune disease - the most common cause in industrialized countries). I would find a half dozen or so hairs in my sink after hair washing and possibly a few hairs on my pillow upon waking but I did not see moderate or severe hair loss. At one point during my thyroid hormone therapy, I was switched from Armour brand, natural thyroid medication to Thyrolar, a synthetic combination T-4/T-3 medication.

After about two weeks on Thyrolar, my hair began to fall out in moderate amounts. I actually was only switched from Armour, to see if mild intermittent hives I was experiencing were due to it but after over a month on Thyrolar, the mild hives continued and so the hives were attributed to my thyroid autoimmunity and not caused by the type thyroid medication I was taking.

With this being the case I asked to be switched back to Armour and the hair loss stopped.

Patients are individuals and none of the scenarios I described are true of everyone. It is also true that most patients taking a type of thyroid medication that does cause them hair loss will see this side effect resolve given additional adjustment time on their thyroid hormone therapy. One importance in the hair loss symptom in people, who are not on thyroid hormone therapy, is recognizing the fact that it can be an indication of thyroid hormone imbalance, especially in people who are experiencing other symptoms that may indicate a change in their thyroid function.

CHAPTER TWO

Diminished Libido

There are many concerning symptoms that can occur with thyroid disease but one of the more concerning ones is loss of libido or a decreased sex drive. One reason this particular symptom can be so concerning is because of the possible strain it can place on the marriage of a thyroid patient (whether real or perceived). I know this concern to be a very real one because I have corresponded with both male and female patients with this problem and concern on thyroid forums, repeatedly over the years since year-2003. It is such a great concern to some of them, that it causes them increased depression symptoms as well.

Patients with more of a problem with loss of libido are those with hypothyroidism. Those with hyperthyroidism can also experience this symptom but they can also experience episodes of increased sex drive, due to the sped up metabolism hyperthyroidism can cause. With hypothyroidism, the metabolism is slowed down, which means the reproductive organs are slowed down as well.

Common Thyroid Disease Complications

The adrenal glands that produce precursor hormones that convert into the sex hormones are also slowed down and both men and women can see decreased testosterone and estrogen levels. Both males and females have both of these sex hormones in their bodies but in different balance for each.

The good news is that when thyroid hormone imbalances of either type are corrected, the result is a normalizing of all bodily functions, including the sex drive. Many thyroid patients report that they regain a certain degree of their libido back although many, report that it is not restored to 100%, as it was before thyroid disease. To regain a significant percentage however is far better than to remain in an almost void state of libido that some patients report.

There are also prescription drugs that can help men in this area and the reason this is slightly more of a concern for men, is due to the fact that they rely upon a bodily function that if not operating properly, prevents intimacy with their partner from taking place.

This fact is also the reason lack of libido can seriously affect some men psychologically because they feel lack of ability to perform sexually, brings into question, their masculinity and ability to satisfy their partner. In some cases, this can then lead them to worry about their marriage in general.

Certainly this is also a concern to women who also have problems with being responsive to their husbands, due to decreased libido. In addition to drugs that can help, there are also hormone therapies that can be administered by a treating Doctor, if the sex hormones are found to be low and in need of additional hormone therapies to correct them.

Thyroid hormone therapy must sometimes be given several months time to help in areas such as libido because it can take this much time to see all bodily organs regain a significant degree of their pre-disease functions. If libido is not adequately restored with thyroid hormone replacement, patients should remember that their Doctors may be able to suggest additional drug or hormone therapies as described above, that can help in this area.

Common Thyroid Disease Complications

CHAPTER THREE

Thyroid Autoimmunity and Hives-Rash (Uticaria)

In recent years, medical research has found a strong connection between thyroid autoimmunity and hives or what is medically known as "chronic uticaria".

Some of the studies specifically state that "Hashimoto's thyroiditis" can be a cause of recurrent hives. Yet even more medical research studies have shown that children with chronic hives or uticaria should be screened for autoimmune thyroid disease by blood testing their thyroid hormone levels and also testing them for "thyroid antibodies".

The two types of thyroid antibodies (also called auto-antibodies), that are most common in causing autoimmune thyroid disease are the "anti-thyroidperoxidase" antibodies (TPO) and the "anti-thyroglobulin" antibodies (TG). If either or both of these are found to be positive in patients with chronic hives, this could be an explanation for their cause.

When I was diagnosed with hypothyroidism, in early 2003, one of the symptoms I experienced that told me something unusual was occurring in my body, was a severe case of hives I experienced, just before worsening symptoms of hypothyroidism, also began to occur.

I had never experienced uticaria previous to this from either allergies or stress and I felt they were a strong indication that something serious was going on with my immune system. It was in fact thyroid auto-immunity that was flaring up in my system and the hives were a result of this chronic immune response that was destroying my thyroid gland and causing me to also experience progressive hypothyroidism (under-active thyroid).

The doctor I visited when the hives were flaring up, felt that I was experiencing a food allergy but this had never happened before and I instead thought it was an allergy to a plant of some type because I had been doing a lot of landscape work at that time, while managing some property. The job I had at the time was also very stressful and so I also considered the severe stress as a possibility.

Common Thyroid Disease Complications

The fact is however that I was experiencing the onset of hypothyroidism, from Hashimoto's thyroiditis.

I feel the disease hit a level of severity, with stress as a possible contributing factor that caused my body to release histamine (fluid produced by the immune system, to fight allergens) which surfaced on my skin, as a severe case of uticaria.

The PubMed medical research website, provided by the National Institutes of Health and the National Library of Medicine, published an article entitled; "Association between chronic urticaria and thyroid autoimmunity: a prospective study involving 99 patients."

The article states the following conclusion; *"This study shows a significant association between chronic urticaria and thyroid autoimmunity, and that tests to detect thyroid autoantibodies are relevant in patients with chronic urticaria, whereas extensive laboratory tests are not."*

When chronic hives (uticaria) is experienced and is an unusual occurrence not easily explained by an allergen or another obvious cause, a patient should see their doctor.

Common Thyroid Disease Complications

They should request thyroid antibodies and thyroid function tests to be ordered. These tests can rule out thyroid autoimmunity or help confirm it as being the cause of this condition.

CHAPTER FOUR

Peripheral Neuropathy

Many thyroid patients complain of neurological type symptoms and many struggle with these despite the fact that they are well treated to correct their thyroid hormone imbalance. In addition to thyroid disorders, other endocrine diseases, such as diabetes can cause symptoms of neuropathy, as can neurological disorders that originate in the brain. "Peripheral Neuropathy" is a term meaning a patient suffers from nerve-related symptoms in their body. These can affect nerves that travel to other parts of the body, so that there is a systemic or referred type effect, meaning there are many areas of the body being affected.

The symptoms of neuropathies can include tingling and numbness sensations in the body but the extremities are more commonly affected (hands and feet). It can also include burning sensations, muscle weakness and stabbing type pains. Muscle twitches and tremor in the muscles can also be a common symptom of peripheral neuropathy (fasciculations).

This particular one affects many thyroid patients with Grave's Disease but can also manifest in those with Hashimoto's thyroiditis.

Some patients with neuropathy type symptoms will also complain of tinnitus, meaning they experience ringing, roaring or clicking sounds in their ears. Some may also experience a degree of hearing loss and dizziness caused by the imbalanced nerve signals reaching the inner ears.

In the year 2007, I had a Brain MRI performed, due to experiencing the symptoms I describe above. My test result came back negative for signs of neurological disease and this confirmed to me that my peripheral neuropathy was likely caused or at least aggravated by my autoimmune thyroid disease.

Some medical sources state that neurological symptoms are rare in thyroid disease patients with hypothyroidism however this is not what I've been hearing from 100s of patients over the years who attest to experiencing neuropathies, despite being well treated.

Common Thyroid Disease Complications

My belief is that these symptoms may originate from thyroid auto-antibody levels and not from thyroid hormone imbalance alone.

There is a severe thyroid antibody condition called "Hashimoto's Encephalitis" (also referred-to as "Hashimoto's Encephalopathy") that causes severe neurological symptoms and is caused by thyroid antibodies (thyroid autoimmunity) however; it is a very rare disorder. It can present with epileptic seizures, amnesia, psychosis and even coma or death.

I feel there are lesser degrees of thyroid antibody related peripheral neuropathy and that it is only common sense to recognize that they can cause neuropathies that are milder than those of Hashimoto's Encephalitis. More on this condition will be addressed in 'CHAPTER FIFTEEN'.

If you are a thyroid patient experiencing peripheral neuropathy symptoms, discuss with your doctor any testing you might need, to rule out causes other than your treated thyroid disease.

Online medical research links that mention Thyroid Disease as a cause of peripheral neuropathy includes the following:

http://www.ninds.nih.gov/disorders/peripheralneuropathy/detail_peripheralneuropathy.htm *(National Institute of Neurological Disorders and Stroke)*

http://www.emedicine.com/neuro/TOPIC214.HTM *(WebMD)*

http://www.pubmedcentral.nih.gov/articlerender.fcgi?artid=1031603 *(PubMed)*

http://www.neurology.org/cgi/content/abstract/67/5/786*(American Academy of Neurology)*

CHAPTER FIVE

Joint and Muscle Pain

Over the past few years, I have corresponded with many thyroid patients with Hashimoto's Disease, the autoimmune type hypothyroidism. Patients with the disease complain of many symptoms they experience with this disease that are caused by antibodies attacking the thyroid gland, causing it to hypo-function but one of the more common ones I hear repeated by patients, is mild to moderate "joint and muscle pain".

This particular symptom is also one of those that can seem to linger in some patients, months or even years after starting treatment for their hypothyroidism, with hormone replacement medication.

Strangely, some patients actually experience a worsening of their joint/muscle pain, once beginning thyroid medication and this was the experience I personally had, after beginning treatment with hormone replacement for Hashimoto's Hypothyroidism.

Common Thyroid Disease Complications

I cannot explain this particular phenomenon but know for a fact, patients do experience it, until their bodies adjust completely to their thyroid medication.

What aspect of this disease, results in the concerning symptoms that affect the patient's joints and muscles? There are many contributing factors however, I believe two of the main causes, are inflammation and decreased blood circulation, from slowed metabolism.

The inflammation aspect is from the autoimmune process that causes antibodies to attack the thyroid gland, resulting in high levels of inflammation. This inflammation first affects the area of the thyroid gland itself but it is my belief, that over time, continuing inflammation is going to eventually have a systemic affect and travel to other parts of the body.

I also believe it is no coincidence that autoimmune disease thyroid patients often complain of their joint pain, first manifesting more severely, in their shoulders and cervical (upper) spine area.

Common Thyroid Disease Complications

These are the joints that are closest to the thyroid. Over time, these joint pains can spread to the other areas of the body, sometimes all the way down to the feet and all the way out to the fingertips.

Inflammation also tends to lead to stiffness in the joints as well, due to mild swelling and fluid around the joints, caused by the release of histamines that are also sent out by the immune system, that act as agents to overwhelm bacterial and viral intruders and reduce inflammation.

Patients with autoimmune thyroid disease, should closely monitor their joint symptoms once on treatment for their hypothyroidism because if they have joint symptoms that result in significant swelling, redness or pain that is more than mild to moderate, this could indicate the onset of Rheumatoid Arthritis (RA), another autoimmune disease, that affects the joints.

There are blood tests that help diagnose or rule out RA specifically, the main one being called "Rheumatoid Factor".

Two others that are sometimes also used in addition to RA Factor are the "ESR" (Erythrocyte Sedimentation Rate), which checks for high levels of inflammation in the body and the "ANA" (Anti-Nuclear Antibodies), which tests for systemic autoimmune disease activity.

One sign a patient can look for their self, is significant swelling and redness in a joint such as a hand, elbow, knee, etc... that is affected equally on both sides of the body. In other words, with Rheumatoid Arthritis, this will manifest in both joints simultaneously, on both sides of the body (symmetrically). Unfortunately, having one autoimmune disease, such as Hashimoto's, places a patient at a higher risk for developing other autoimmune disorders and is why this joint pain aspect should be monitored closely if rheumatic symptoms are occurring.

The mild to moderate muscle pain (rheumatic or fibromyalgic pain), in hypothyroidism which can include cramping and spasms, in my belief, is due to a slowing down of all organs in the body, due to lack of thyroid hormone, which also regulates our metabolism.

Common Thyroid Disease Complications

This causes blood circulation to become less adequate and so the muscles are not nourished by blood and oxygen as they should be.

Strangely, some hypothyroid patients experience hypertension (high blood pressure) because the disease causes blood vessels to constrict but at the same time, they do not have proper blood circulation to some of their muscles because heart function is slightly reduced due to slowed metabolism. This affect, also causes symptoms in tendons and ligaments and many hypothyroid patients also complain of "Carpal Tunnel Syndrome" (hand/wrist) and "Tarsal Tunnel Syndrome" (feet).

If a patient has severe, ongoing muscle symptoms, they should seek further medical testing, as I also recommended for joint pain patients, to rule out possible Muscle Disease and Connective Tissue Diseases. Some of the same tests as mentioned above are used to help diagnose muscle disease but there are others as well, such as one called "Anti-Smooth Muscle Antibodies".

There are many Connective Tissue Diseases, including "Lupus" and some patients can experience "Overlap Syndromes", meaning they are experiencing more than one type.

A well-informed doctor is important when you are being treated for autoimmune hypothyroidism, one who understands the risks for other autoimmune disease disorders and one who can detect when symptoms may indicate something other than thyroid related ones. I have visited a few doctors in the past who actually did not know that hypothyroidism caused joint and muscle pain.

I have also known of other doctors who did not recognize emotional symptoms as being thyroid related in patients they were treating but actually believe these were separate issues. This is why a truly good, caring, well informed doctor is worth her/his weight in gold!

In conclusion I would like to add that many times, these mild to moderate joint pain symptoms, can be treated with over-the-counter anti-inflammatory medications.

There are also very effective over-the-counter, natural supplements that help with joint pain and inflammation, one of these being a combination of "Glucosamine and Chondroitin". It is also very important to take your thyroid medication as recommended by your Physician and let him/her know about other supplements you may choose to take in addition to your hormone replacement.

If it takes a prescription strength medication to treat your joint/muscle pain symptoms, it might be time to ask your doctor for further testing.

CHAPTER SIX

Fatigue Despite Thyroid Hormone Therapy?

The first thing I always suggest to treated hypothyroid patients who experience low energy and fatigue that is an important consideration when being replaced with thyroid hormone, is making sure the hormone therapy is being as optimized as possible.

Some doctors only treat to get the TSH level anywhere within the normal range but some patients need a TSH that is really suppressed, in order to feel better. The low normal at most labs for TSH is from about 0.3 to 0.5 and some patients need theirs to be at these lowest normal levels to see significant symptom relief and a doctor willing to work with them in trials of doses that get them there.

If you haven't received copies of labs you've had done to monitor your thyroid hormone therapy, I would ask for your most recent ones, to see where your doctor has put your TSH level (the "HIPPA" law in the U.S. grants patient's copies).

If he has kept your TSH level at above 2.0 especially, you need to discuss a trial of a dose that will suppress the level down to below a 1.0 or even lower-normal.

Some doctors are overly concerned that getting TSH that low will cause hyperthyroid symptoms however this won't happen with close monitoring and with also testing the Free T-3 and Free T-4 levels for better monitoring of a dose that suppresses your TSH.

Other than this, I like to suggest a good multi-vitamin to thyroid patients but especially ones with B-12 and the other B vitamins because these help with energy. The sublingual type (liquid, i.e. "Perfect B" Brand) is good because it absorbs quickly and can be taken twice daily to help maintain energy levels through the day.

Some patients also report better symptom relief and improved energy levels by cutting wheat and dairy from their diet as well (takes discipline). This is due to the fact that glutton intolerance (sensitivity to wheat products) is more common in autoimmune thyroid patients.

Common Thyroid Disease Complications

Dairy products can flare the symptoms of lactose intolerance in thyroid patients as well. Both conditions have potential to negatively affect energy levels in the body.

These are suggestions that can aid thyroid hormone therapy in relieving hypothyroid symptoms, including low energy and fatigue, the best possible.

CHAPTER SEVEN

Is Dysautonomia Common in Thyroid Patients?

"Dysautonoma", is one of those disorders that is similar in recognition to CFS, Fibromyalgia and adrenal fatigue, being a disorder that comes in several types, that like these others is not known about or recognized by many Doctors, although it is gaining recognition. There are a very real group of disorders that are in the dysautonomia category, recognized and described in detail, on the most reputable medical sources, including the National Institutes of Health.

Dysautonomia disorders cause dysfunction of the involuntary nervous system at different levels of severity, also called the "autonomic nervous system". This is the part of our nervous system that regulates involuntary bodily functions such as heart rate, respiration, liver function, kidney function, adrenal function, etc.... Some of these functions you might think we control but actually we can only influence them because when you sleep, heart beat and breathing continues, as do these other involuntary bodily functions.

Common Thyroid Disease Complications

Some types of dysautonomia, are more commonly found in thyroid patients, such as Mitral Valve Prolapse Syndrome (some medical sites add "dysautonomia" into the MVPS title). While the Mitral Valve Prolapse itself, is a heart murmur, caused by looseness or thickness of the mitral valve leaflets in the heart, many reputable medical sources state that people who actually have symptoms from it, have a co-morbid dysautonomia with it. They actually do not know if MVP causes dysautonomia in some patients or if the co-existence of dysautonomia with MVP is what causes more symptoms (syndrome). I personally believe the latter theory is the one that is more likely.

Another very common form of dysautonomia is "orthostatic hypotension", also referred to as "postural hypotention". This one causes you to feel faint, due to a blood pressure drop upon standing from a seated or lying down position (supine positions) and it is also sometimes referred to as "neurally mediated hypotension" (NMH). This form of dysautonomia is also found in conditions such as CFS, Fibromyalgia and conditions that affect adrenal function.

They also do not know if this type dysautonomia, with broader aspects to it, is the cause of these syndromes or just part of the manifestations of them.

There is a medical test for this one, called the "tilt-table test", which consists of taking a patient's blood pressure and heart rate readings, when sitting or lying flat, then again when at various upright positions. I have this type of dysautonomia and would be revealed clearly if I were to have this tilt-table test done. You can do a home-version of this test yourself using a BP monitor, by first taking a reading while sitting, then again immediately upon standing to monitor for abnormal changes.

When I do this test at home, my BP drops a good 20 points and my heart rate increases 30 or more BPM. This is too much of a fluctuation and an overreaction by the involuntary nervous system, which would also be revealed via a tilt-table test and points to an involuntary nervous system that is struggling to regulate these bodily functions (dysregulated-autonomic "dys-autonomia").

The treatment for OH is usually simple lifestyle changes, when it is mild to moderate, including exercise and eating healthy, making sure there is ample salt in the diet and drinking plenty of water which all help to keep low blood pressure episodes from happening (hypotension). When drug therapy for OH is used, it may include "Fludrocortisone" (Florinef), a mineral corticosteroid used to help regulate blood pressure, Midodrine (alpha-1 adrenergic agonist), Methylphenidate (amphetamine) and Ephedrine (adrenaline). These drug treatments are not recommended or prescribed however, when lifestyle and diet changes are able to control OH.

I have had this form of dysautonomia, since childhood but much worse since experiencing the onset of autoimmune thyroid disease. Interestingly, I was also diagnosed with a heart murmur, at age 14 or 15 and an MD and a Cardiologist, both thought it was "Wolf-Parkinson-White Syndrome" (a more serious heart murmur) but a modern-day cardiologist ruled it out and I now know they were detecting MVP in me because much less was know about it and dysautonomia in the 1970s.

If a patient suspects they have a form of dysautonomia, they should discuss this with their Doctor. The patient might then be referred to a specialist who is familiar with the group of disorders that come under this heading. These include; Postural Orthostatic Tachycardia Syndrome (POTS), Neurocardiogenic Syncope, Mitral Valve Prolapse Dysautonomia, Pure Autonomic Failure, Multiple System Atrophy (Shy-Drager syndrome), Autonomic Instability and other less severe types including Orthostatic Hypotension, which can manifest alone or as a feature of one of these others or syndromes that may also include it as a feature.

Dysautonomia can be a mild condition or severe and even life-threatening and so it is important that patients, who suspect they have it, are diagnosed and treated.

CHAPTER EIGHT

Anxiety, Panic and Depression

If you have thyroid disease, you may have experienced some co-morbid (related) anxiety along with it.

This can especially be true if you have autoimmune thyroid disease, which includes Graves' Disease/hyperthyroidism and Hashimoto's thyroiditis, which can cause Hashitoxicosis (intermittent hyperthyroidism).

A very unpleasant type of anxiety reaction is one called "panic attacks" and if you experience them frequently, it is referred to as "Panic Disorder". These are very unpleasant anxiety attacks that cause anxiety symptoms to escalate suddenly.

When people experience them, they will often hyperventilate and experience a racing heart and an extreme fear emotion. This article is intended to show you that you are far from being alone in experiencing these.

Panic Disorder Description and Statistics

"Panic Attacks" are what you might describe as the "climax of anxiety" and are truly unpleasant, to say the least, as we who have experienced them know! They can occur with just about any other anxiety disorder, including Generalized Anxiety Disorder (GAD) but when the panic attacks themselves are the feature-manifestation, it is referred to as "Panic Disorder" (PD). They can hit extremely hard and a person first experiencing them will commonly believe they are having a heart attack.

Many people new to the panic attack experience find their selves in hospital emergency rooms, only to be told everything physically checks out normal, once they return to a calmed state. Many new to the panic experience will also believe they are going mad/insane or that another attack will cause them to completely lose control.

Approximately 6 million American adults ages 18 and older, or about 2.7 percent of people in this age group in a given year, have panic disorder. Panic disorder typically develops in early adulthood (median age of onset is 24).

However, the age of onset can extend throughout adulthood. About one in three people with panic disorder develops agoraphobia, a condition in which the individual becomes afraid of being in any place or situation where escape might be difficult or help unavailable in the event of a panic attack (statistics by the National Institute of Mental Health, reprints allowed for public education).

Hypothyroid Therapy and Anxiety/Depression

What is really important when a thyroid patient is being treated for hypothyroidism is that they are on optimal dose of "thyroid hormone replacement therapy medication" (HRT). When a patient is placed on a dose of HRT, most will need 1, 2 or 3 dose changes (usually increases) before they reach the adequate/optimal level.

When some Doctors place a patient on thyroid hormone and if that first dose gets their thyroid blood lab levels, anywhere into the normal range, they simply stop there. They do not afterward try to "optimize" the patient's HRT.

Some patients need more of a targeted treatment goal, for example, many patients do not see symptoms resolve significantly, unless their dose gets their "TSH" level (most common thyroid lab test Doctors use to monitor HRT), at about "1.0" and some may even need their TSH level at lowest normal, which is about "0.3 to 0.5". A Doctor has to be willing to work with a patient in getting their HRT optimized, by going by their symptoms as well as their lab levels.

In regard to emotional symptoms caused by thyroid disease, anxiety and depression are commonly listed and patients not being treated optimally may see these symptoms linger. Some do also need the addition of antidepressant and anti-anxiety medications but some patients see their emotional symptoms resolve with thyroid HRT alone.

In my case as a hypothyroid patient, once I was treated on the correct dose of thyroid HRT, my emotional symptoms of anxiety and depression resolved within a couple of months. Previous to this however, I was treated by a different doctor who did not optimize my HRT.

Common Thyroid Disease Complications

I struggled with anxiety and depressive symptoms for nearly two years. That doctor kept my TSH between 3.0 and 5.0 and I'm the type patient that needs a very low TSH (lowest normal). Not all patients need a lowest-normal TSH to see symptom relief but a good target range to start with, is the "1.0" I mention above.

Some Doctors will claim that depression and anxiety are not caused by hypothyroidism but it certainly is, especially the autoimmune type-Hashimoto's (type I have) and many research studies have concluded this. Almost all reputable medical sources list "depression" as a symptom of hypothyroidism and many have added "anxiety" to the list as well.

Patients should be pro-active in discussing optimal HRT with their Doctors because it is after all a person's health at stake, which affects every aspect of their lives.

It is only right that hypothyroid patients be treated, so that they can pursue their livelihood, family needs and enjoyment and all around quality of life.

There are sensational Doctors out there but the ones, who don't understand the need to optimally treat hypothyroid patients, in my opinion, should refer their hypothyroid patients, to the Doctors who do believe in thyroid HRT optimization.

CHAPTER NINE

Metabolic Related Complications

Hypothyroidism and Fatty Liver Disease

As I mention in other articles, people with one metabolic disorder, including thyroid disease, are at higher risk for developing other metabolic disorders and diseases. For example, a patient with hypothyroidism is at increased risk for developing Metabolic Syndrome (a pre-diabetes syndrome), Adult Onset Diabetes and Adrenal Syndromes/Diseases. This is especially true if the thyroid disease they have is the autoimmune type.

Another metabolic related condition that can occur in thyroid patients, as well as in a large percent of the population is one called "Non-Alcoholic Fatty Liver Disease" (NAFLD). This disease is metabolic related due to the fact that the body is storing an excessive amount of fat in this major organ called the liver, rather than converting more of it into energy needed by the body.

Common Thyroid Disease Complications

One reason this happens is due to over-consumption of fats and sugars, combined with being overweight and the inability of the liver to keep up with the demand for conversion of these into energy.

When the liver becomes overwhelmed in this performance of duty, it instead begins to store more fat. Over time, this causes mild inflammation in the liver and liver cell damage (hepatic response or "steatosis hepatitis") and over time can actually cause lesions in the liver or "liver sclerosis". While most cases of fatty liver do not lead to actual hepatitis or sclerosis, it is a risk people with fatty liver should be aware of, so that they can undertake diet and lifestyle changes, in order to keep the condition under control and to possibly resolve or reverse it over time.

Most cases of fatty liver disease are caused by alcohol consumption and since this type I'm addressing in this article is not, the "non-alcoholic" prefix is used. It is true however that despite the fact it is not alcohol related, people with the non-alcoholic type are highly advised to avoid alcohol consumption.

Common Thyroid Disease Complications

What are some other ways to help control and possibly resolve NAFLD that some statistics state may affect up to one-third of the population? Well, as is recommended for most metabolic disorders and diseases, patients need to incorporate a healthy regimen of exercise and weight loss/control into their schedules. Even if this means simply walking for 20 minutes at least three times per week.

Patients should also avoid fatty foods and refined sugars which both can be stored as fat in the liver. Eating more fruits and vegetables and foods containing lots of fiber can also help with this disease. It is also important to lose weight when you are carrying extra pounds, especially that that accumulates in the mid-section of the body.

Most people have no physical symptoms of this disease although the most common symptoms reported are fatigue and dull pain on the right side, just under the rib cage. NAFLD is usually found incidentally when a patient is blood tested and the tests include a metabolic panel that includes liver function tests. Their liver enzymes will be mildly to moderately, elevated (ALT and SGPT or AST levels).

Once these abnormal liver counts are found, an ultrasound imaging of the liver is performed to confirm fatty infiltration of the liver.

If you are a thyroid disease patient, or one that has Metabolic Syndrome or Diabetes, a "Metabolic Panel" including liver function tests should be performed via blood testing, once a year, to detect possible development of fatty liver disease. If this disorder is detected a Doctor may prescribe a treatment plan similar to the one I describe above but medications may also be prescribed in more severe cases.

Hypothyroidism and Metabolic Syndrome

There are many co-morbid disorders that can affect thyroid patients. One of those is a syndrome affecting the body's metabolism, called "Metabolic Syndrome".

According to reputable medical sources, this syndrome affects millions of people and puts them at higher risk for developing diabetes, heart disease and other potentially serious health problems.

This syndrome has gained recognition because of its ability to significantly increase the risk for diabetes and in past years was known by other names including "Syndrome X".

Medical research conclusions link the Metabolic Syndrome to thyroid dysfunction, some including the link listed below (type into your PC browser to view), associate it with "sub-clinical hypothyroidism". What I feel is significant about this study is the fact that most hypothyroid patients who are later treated, experienced long standing sub-clinical hypothyroidism, before progressing to overt (full blown) hypothyroidism. This means most of us who were diagnosed with hypothyroidism, were at risk for Metabolic Syndrome.

Link>
http://jcem.endojournals.org/cgi/content/abstract/jc.2006-1718v1 (Journal of Clinical Endocrinology & Metabolism)

Metabolic Syndrome occurs when a person gains extra weight and has become less active, so that their bodies lack the needed exercise to help them burn fat and calories.

Common Thyroid Disease Complications

The hormone in the body that aids in this process is "insulin". This pancreatic hormone takes glucose, fats and carbohydrates (sugar, starch, cellulose) and helps to convert them into energy that is needed by the body. Glucose is essential in the body and without it, the body cannot function.

A major organ that depends highly upon glucose is the brain. When someone who is at risk for developing Metabolic Syndrome due to being overweight and inactive consumes fats, sugars and carbohydrates, their bodies begin to store these rather than burn them off or convert them into energy. The lack of glucose metabolism is referred to as "Insulin Resistance".

Over time, insulin resistance can evolve into Type II Diabetes or what is also referred to as Adult Onset Diabetes. In addition to this syndrome increasing the risk of diabetes, it can also contribute to hypertension, elevated cholesterol and heart disease.

Other medical sources also associate Metabolic Syndrome with Non-Alcoholic Fatty Liver Disease (NAFLD).

The symptoms that indicate development of this syndrome include; weight gain, especially in the mid-section of your body, development of hypertension, hypoglycemic episodes (lows in glucose energy levels before and after meals), mood swings and inability to concentrate (brain fog). People, who are developing this disorder, will often have borderline diabetic glucose levels, when they are blood lab tested for diabetes. They will also often have elevated cholesterol and triglyceride levels.

Improving your diet by eliminating refined sugars, cutting back on unhealthy fats (saturated/trans fats) and simple carbohydrates (pies, cakes, candies & soft drinks) and eating more complex carbohydrates (fruits vegetables, nuts & grains) plus keeping your weight down and exercising will significantly reduce your chances of developing Metabolic Syndrome and the serious health complications that can develop from it.

Thyroid patients with hypothyroidism are at increased risk for other metabolic disorders, such as diabetes as well as this pre-diabetes condition called Metabolic Syndrome.

Common Thyroid Disease Complications

Preventing Diabetes in Thyroid Patients

Type 2 Diabetes is also called Adult Onset Diabetes and affects an estimated 15-million Americans. It is more common in adults ages 45 and over and more common in people with other endocrine disorders, including thyroid diseases. There are steps that can be taken to reduce your risk of experiencing the onset of this disease that causes a dysfunction in the way your body metabolizes your blood sugar (glucose), as outlined below.

Avoid weight gain and excessively high blood glucose, by being faithful to a diet low in refined sugars. Refined sugars are those that do not come naturally but are processed sugars used to manufacture junk foods, such as cakes, cookies, candies, pies and soft drinks. Consuming too much refined sugar not only causes excess weight gain but over time, can also cause the body to lose its ability to regulate that sugar via the hormone called insulin. This hormone that is released by the pancreas, helps metabolize (convert) the sugar we consume, into energy for the body and helps carry that energy to every cell in the body.

Without adequate glucose in the blood, our organs do not function properly and one major organ that is highly dependent upon glucose is the brain as previously mentioned. There is however a limit to how much glucose the body is able to metabolize and when there is a continual excess of it, it is converted into fat and carbohydrates as well and stored in the body.

Over time, this causes weight gain and an inability of the body to continue converting the excess amounts of glucose being consumed and at this point, a person may develop a condition called "insulin resistance", a pre-diabetic condition that over time has the potential to become full blown diabetes.

Incorporate adequate exercise into your weekly schedule, which helps to keep your weight down and helps the body to metabolize glucose. Exercise is essential in helping to burn calories and fat in the body, so that less of it is stored. Exercise also helps the body to build muscle tissue from the things we eat, rather than inactivity, which contributes to the body storing more fat.

It also helps the body by circulating the hormones that are active in the blood stream and that contribute to our health, energy and metabolism, including insulin, which regulates our blood glucose levels. Even mild exercise such as walking for 20 minutes, three or more times a week, can help the body with metabolism and prevention of weight gain and can contribute to weight loss.

Get regular check ups by your Doctor and monitor your glucose levels regularly, especially if diabetes runs in your family. It is a good idea for everyone to get yearly check ups by their Doctor but if one or both of your parents or one of your siblings has diabetes, this becomes even more important. Diabetes, like other endocrine diseases (glandular), can run in families and so if a close relative has diabetes, you are at significantly increased risk for developing the disease yourself.

Early prevention is the key to avoiding this potentially serious disease, which upon experiencing the onset of, also puts a person at higher risk for heart disease, kidney failure and glaucoma.

Common Thyroid Disease Complications

Glaucoma is an eye disorder that can eventually lead to diminished eyesight and even blindness.

Home glucose monitors are available, that allow a person to check their own blood glucose levels regularly, in the convenience of their home. A person at risk for diabetes can check their glucose level at different times of the day and keep a record of their readings, so that they can detect any pattern or change in their glucose regulation and report these changes to their Doctor.

Avoid alcohol or only consume it in cautious moderation. People at risk for diabetes or who actually have diabetes are cautioned to avoid alcohol if possible or to at least drink it in moderation. Alcohol reacts very quickly in the body and your body depends on your liver to clear the alcohol from your system because it is recognized by the body as a toxin.

When you drink alcohol, the liver will not function in converting glucose into carbohydrates and fat because it is busy clearing the body of alcohol and this, results in a spike or increase in glucose levels in the blood.

People who are on insulin shots to treat their diabetes or on an oral medication can seriously hinder the effectiveness of their medication, through alcohol consumption and this is especially true when they consume alcohol on an empty stomach or in excessive amounts.

The liver and the hormone insulin, both work in the body to regulate glucose, the liver being the organ that converts it into fat and carbohydrates or "stored energy" and insulin being the hormone that converts it into "immediate energy" for the cells of the body.

Treated Hypothyroidism and Weight Gain

It is a well known fact that untreated hypothyroidism causes moderate weight gain, in fact some patients report weight gain that is in excess of moderate.

I use the term moderate however, because most medical sources state it that way and they also suggest that weight gain with untreated hypothyroidism will usually result in no more than 20lb of weight gain.

Regardless of the actual amount of weight gain, which in my opinion varies among individual patients and depends upon how severe their untreated hypothyroidism is, it does indeed cause weight gain! This is due to the fact that with hypothyroid conditions, the rate of our bodily metabolism is slowed down. We burn less energy when the metabolism is not running at a normal rate. They also refer to this as hypo-metabolism, which can have additional causes other than hypothyroidism.

Now when we look at patients who are being treated for hypothyroidism, we still hear them report gaining weight more easily and having difficulty losing weight. There are no medical research studies on the subject of weight gain in patients being treated for hypothyroidism that I am aware of but the number of patients attesting to this problem in articles and on forums is significant. I personally can also attest to the fact that I too gain weight more easily and have a harder time losing weight, despite being adequately and even optimally treated for my hypothyroidism.

I'm not sure we will ever have a firm medical explanation as to why this happens but it could possibly be that thyroid hormone being administered from the outside (hormone therapy), whether it is the natural or synthetic form, is slightly less effective in regulating our metabolism than our own hormone is. This is certainly just a theory but in my opinion, is a reasonable one that should be given some consideration by those in the medical profession.

Another theory that I believe should be considered, is the possibility that "thyroid autoimmunity" that is present in most cases of hypothyroidism, may also play a factor in weight control. It may be that thyroid antibodies also affect our metabolism, to a very small degree but significant enough to affect our body's ability to burn calories and turn fat into energy. I do know that "insulin resistance" is more common in treated hypothyroid patients and the description I just gave, fits this condition. I can also attest to being a hypothyroid patient with co-morbid insulin resistance.

Treated hypothyroid patients must work harder than people without thyroid disease, to lose weight and to keep their weight under control. While there are many diet plans out there, I feel the same principles apply in weight loss, no matter which diet plan you may try.

The principles include eating healthier, which would consist of eating more fruits, vegetables, nuts and grains, cutting back and eliminating refined sugars from your diet, eating less and exercising more. These principles can be wrapped together in many different packages and called by many different diet-plan names but they are the principles that work and you simply add discipline to that plan, to make it work.

Weight gain and difficulty losing weight is a challenge to treated hypothyroid patients but one they can accomplish with effort.

CHAPTER TEN

Thyroid Eye Disease

Graves' Ophthalmology (GO) is a co-occurring inflammatory condition affecting the eyes (also called Thyroid Eye Disease). Some medical sources state that GO is present to varied degrees in 50% of Graves' disease patients (those with autoimmune hyperthyroidism) but only requires corrective surgical procedures in approximately 5% of cases.

This means it can potentially develop in up to half of Grave's patients and rarely a type of this condition can also develop in patients with Hashimoto's thyroiditis (in about 2% of patients with autoimmune hypothyroidism).

It can also cause bulging of the eyes (proptosis) and possible deterioration of vision. The duration of symptoms can occur for 1 to 3 years before they resolve through the natural course of the disease and/or through treatments, if necessary and depending on the severity of its manifestation.

The most common treatments for GO/Thyroid Eye Disease include:

• *Eye drops to keep the eyes lubricated*

• *Corticosteroid therapy (steroid anti-inflammatory)*

• *Radiotherapy and/or Decompression Therapy to reduce orbital damage*

• *Eyelid surgery to lengthen eyelids that may not cover the eyes well due to them bulging*

• GD patients who smoke are sometimes also given the recommendation by their doctors to quit smoking because of the inflammatory chemicals contained in cigarettes that can potentially affect the eyes.

(TED) can cause serious damage and even blindness in some patients. Unfortunately, with regard to Graves ' disease, patients who do develop Graves' Ophthalmology (GO), treatment for the condition may not be able to prevent eye damage even though they are already well treated for their hyperthyroidism.

CHAPTER ELEVEN

Adrenal Fatigue and Thyroid Patients

A lot of us with thyroid disease also have some co-existing adrenal fatigue and in fact have been discussing this quite a bit on some of the thyroid forums and message boards for a number of years.

Add to thyroid disease, something like a traumatic or very stressful even and you can really suffer from adrenal fatigue. Your circadian rhythms are off with this condition and are why your sleep patterns are disrupted. Your cortisol and DHEA will have their peaks, at the wrong times, such as at sleep time and your normal drop in these hormones also happens at the wrong time, like during the day, when you most need the peak energy. Adrenal fatigue that goes on for a long time (chronic) then becomes "adrenal exhaustion" and this is the point to where you no longer experience those needed peak levels at all.

I have had adrenal fatigue for several years, as a feature of Chronic Fatigue Syndrome and have also experienced adrenal exhaustion.

Mine turned into adrenal exhaustion, after experiencing the onset of Hashimoto's/hypothyroidism and at the same time, I had gone through a terribly stressful period of time (chronic stressors).

Mine did not improve when I first began thyroid hormone replacement but actually worsened for a time. After several months on the correct thyroid dose, I finally saw some improvement in thyroid and adrenal symptoms but at times of extra stress and extended periods of hard physical activity, I've taken some adrenal support supplements that I learned about when researching about adrenal fatigue. These included multi "B" vitamins, especially B-12, in sublingual form (liquid) and vitamin "C", magnesium, selenium, zinc, DHEA 25mg (an over-the-counter adrenal hormone) and sometimes but less often, an Adrenal Cortex Extract (processed beef adrenal glands in pill form).

These always help me a great deal but I don't supplement with the ones containing actual adrenal hormone, as a permanent regimen.

However, as safe as they are at the recommended doses, it would not hurt for me to do so, according to research that has been conducted on these supplements.

I seriously considered Cortef (natural adrenal steroid) and had a Dr. willing to treat me with it but I was just a little wary of steroids and I still am. I have however, read many reputable medical resources that state that Cortef is safe as physiological doses (25mg and less), to supplement a person's low cortisol levels from adrenal exhaustion but can cause "adrenal suppression", if administered in full replacement doses (above 25mg) and if used for extended periods. In my opinion, adrenal support supplements are usually all that is needed for most cases of adrenal fatigue.

How does a patient know if they have adrenal fatigue? Blood adrenal hormone levels can be helpful but are like a "snapshot reading" and since cortisol levels go up when you are stressed, like at a blood draw, this can affect the snapshot blood level.

This is why saliva testing is recommended because you can conveniently get several readings over a 24 hour period to establish the adrenal hormone rhythms.

Saliva testing has been researched and found very accurate, in fact it is used to monitor hormone levels in medical research, including that done by the World Health Organizations. It is also an approved form of testing, by many major health insurance companies, such as Blue Cross/Blue Shield.

Many pharmacies carry the type manufactured by "ZRT Labs, Inc.", which is also a U.S. approved blood lab, so you might check with your pharmacy to see if they carry this brand, if you suspect adrenal fatigue is affecting you.

Most adrenal saliva tests are not really expensive and can be diagnostic in detecting adrenal fatigue.

While the above list of thyroid disease complications does not include all of them, these are some of the major ones that are experienced. See your doctor for further evaluation and treatment options.

Common Thyroid Disease Complications

CHAPTER TWELVE

What are Goiters?

When a thyroid patient has a goiter, this simply means they have swelling of the thyroid gland, which is located at the front of the neck, in the area just below the Adam's apple. Goiters are recognized as different types and as affecting part of the thyroid, such as one of the two lobes (one on each side of the gland) or the middle part of the gland called the isthmus or as affecting the entire gland as a whole. They are also considered different types depending upon the causes of them.

How Goiters are Detected/Diagnosed

Patients, who have goiters or are suspected of having them, may be referred for a "thyroid ultrasound" (sound-wave imaging/sonogram) or "thyroid uptake scan" (radiology/radioactive iodine) and possibly even an MRI (Magnetic Resonance Imaging).

These are diagnostic tests that give detailed images of the thyroid gland, to determine the size of goiters and whether they contain nodules within them that are not detectable by palpation.

Types of Goiters

A major cause of goiters, are autoimmune thyroid diseases. If a person's thyroid gland has swelling plus a number of small tumors called "nodules" within it, they refer to this type as a "multi-nodular goiter". The nodules within a gland that has goiter can be the type that causes the thyroid gland to produce excess thyroid hormone, in which case, they will add the term "toxic" to the term, calling it a "toxic multi-nodular goiter".

People with Hashimoto's thyroiditis, commonly have multi-nodular goiters that are non- toxic. When a person is termed as having a "diffuse goiter", this means there is general swelling throughout the gland that is not caused by nodules. This type of goiter can also cause toxicity or over-activity of the thyroid gland (hyperthyroidism), in which case it is referred to as a "toxic diffuse goiter".

Common Thyroid Disease Complications

These types are found commonly in patients with Grave's Disease, as well as toxic multi-nodular goiters.

If a goiter is caused by iodine deficiency, it is referred to as a "colloid nodular" or "endemic' goiter. This type is rare in the U.S. and many other industrialized countries that use iodized table salt, which usually provides those that consume it, enough iodine to avoid iodine deficiency hypothyroidism and the resulting endemic goiters.

Temporary types of thyroiditis, such as those that occur with viral infections and in pregnant women can also cause goiter (asymmetrical enlargement) but these type will resolve within a few weeks, along with the thyroiditis. These type goiters can flare up short term with these types of thyroiditis and cause severe pain in the thyroid gland, which is referred to as "sub-acute thyroiditis", while others types do not cause a painful thyroid which is referred to as "silent thyroiditis".

CHAPTER THIRTEEN

What are Thyroid Nodules?

Thyroid nodules are small tumor-like growths on the thyroid gland. According to statistics, as much as 10 percent of the population has thyroid nodules but they occur far more often in thyroid diseases. People with autoimmune thyroid diseases have abnormal thyroid tissue and over time can develop a large number of nodules or what is referred to as "multi-nodules".

How Thyroid Nodules are Detected/Diagnosed

Thyroid nodules can be detected by feel or "palpation" but some may be in an area of the gland that are only detectable by diagnostic imaging tests such as "thyroid ultrasound" (sound wave imaging), "Radio Active Iodine Uptake Scans" (radiological imaging) and "MRI" (Magnetic Resonance Imaging).

Thyroid nodules that are solitary or found to be a single one, rather than found among a group of them have a slightly higher risk of containing cancer cells (malignancy) than do multi-nodules.

Larger nodules are also considered more suspicious. When a solitary nodule is located, the treating Doctor may wish to have a tissue biopsy performed.

The procedure that is usually performed to obtain a thyroid nodule tissue sample is called a "Fine Needle Aspiration" (FNA) and is a simple out-patient procedure. The tissue sample is then lab-analyzed to detect any abnormal cells indicating the presence of either "papillary" or "follicular" cancer, which are the two major types that can potentially invade the thyroid gland.

Types of Thyroid Nodules

When thyroid nodules are being investigated, they may be placed into several categories. Two of the more basic categories of thyroid nodules, are those that are solitary (single ones) and multi-nodules (a group of several) but other terms used in describing them include "hot nodules", meaning the nodule is actively absorbing iodine from the thyroid gland and is releasing thyroid hormone, causing a hormone imbalance in the patient (hyperthyroidism).

Smaller hot nodules may not cause hyperthyroidism while larger ones usually do and many times are also biopsied due to their larger size. If the nodule is not causing thyroid hormone release, it is referred to as a "cold nodule" and both hot and cold nodules have a distinct appearance on diagnostic imaging tests.

Some thyroid nodules are more solid than others which are referred to as a "solid nodules" and these are also considered more suspicious of possibly containing cancer cells and may also be biopsied as a precaution, depending upon their size. Many non-solid nodules are considered to be "cystic nodules" because they will contain fluid in the center of them and these type, are almost never considered a risk for containing cancer cells.

Treatment for Goiters and Thyroid Nodules

The most common treatment for both goiters and benign thyroid nodules is thyroid hormone replacement therapy. Treating doctors will prescribe a dose of thyroid hormone that can help to shrink goiters and nodules over time and can also prevent further growth of them.

Common Thyroid Disease Complications

If a goiter or thyroid nodule is large enough to obstruct a patient's breathing or swallowing, a treating doctor might refer the patient for surgery, to remove a nodule or part of the thyroid gland and possibly all of the thyroid gland.

In cases of malignancy found in the thyroid gland, total thyroid removal is always the treatment. Afterward the patient must have thyroid hormone replacement therapy for the rest of their lives. More in regard to malignant thyroid conditions will be discussed in the next segments addressing thyroid cancer.

CHAPTER FOURTEEN

Thyroid Cancer a Less Common Thyroid Disease Manifestation

Of all the thyroid disorders and diseases that are out there, thyroid cancer is the least common of all of them but at the same time is also increasing faster than any other form of cancer.

Thyroid cancer should be taken very seriously as should any form of cancer because any type that is not caught in time and treated has the potential to spread to other parts of the body.

According to medical research on thyroid cancer, chances of developing it are increased in people with a family history of thyroid cancer.

At the same time, thyroid cancer has a very high treatment success rate and that success rate is increased when early diagnosis and treatment is started. According to medical sources, only about 5% of thyroid nodules are found to contain cancer.

How Thyroid Cancer Manifests

Thyroid cancers always present as thyroid nodules (tumors) in the thyroid gland but some tumors are more easily recognizable than others. In the case of thyroid nodules, an FNA (tissue biopsy) of these may be necessary, when they are of a certain size that makes them suspicious of possibly containing malignancy or cancer cells. The same is true if nodules are found to be solid, meaning they are not typical nodules that are softer in texture (warm nodules) or cystic but are very firm, which are also sometimes referred to as "cold nodules".

Single nodules are also considered more suspicious than are multi-nodules, meaning several of them, rather than a single one and might also have FNA biopsies ordered to evaluate them. While an FNA can detect certain types of cancers that affect the thyroid gland, other types, such as carcinomas need surgical biopsies performed to detect them. More about the FNA test will be discussed in the next segment in regard to diagnosing thyroid cancer.

Some types of thyroid cancer tumors, take on the appearance of thyroid gland tissue which means they are less malignant and more treatable. The type, that resemble thyroid tissue are referred to as "differentiated". Other types have a distinctly different appearance from normal thyroid tissue and these types are referred to as "undifferentiated" and have a higher malignancy and are more difficult to treat successfully.

Many thyroid tumors (nodules) are found incidentally, when a person happens to detect one by feel or they may feel a lump on the inside of their throat when swallowing. When the patient sees their doctor, he may palpate (feel) the nodule to see if it feels firm or of significant size. If he finds that the nodule needs further investigation, he may refer the patient for testing.

Sometimes, a thyroid nodule will grow toward the inside of the throat, and the person will feel it as a lump when swallowing. If the nodule is malignant, and it is an aggressive type of cancer, the nodule can grow large enough to obstruct breathing and swallowing.

How Thyroid Cancer is Diagnosed

There are a number of procedures used to diagnose thyroid cancer, including blood tests to detect levels of thyroglobulin, cancer cells (new advancements) and for the presence of "Calcitonin" (found with medullary cancer). Imaging tests may also be ordered, including a Thyroid Ultrasound, CT Scans, MRIs and 24 hour Thyroid Uptake Scans.

The single most diagnostic test to detect the presence of thyroid cancer, are biopsies of the affected thyroid tissue. This includes using a fine needle to extract tissue samples (Fine Needle Biopsy) and surgical biopsies when needed.

An FNA is performed using a needle that is inserted into the patient's thyroid gland and tissue from the gland or nodules being biopsied, is extracted and sent for laboratory analysis. While it is a fairly non-evasive procedure, patients should expect some soreness for a few days following the procedure. The fine needle that is used does not leave scarring and a local anesthesia is used to numb the area on the neck, before the needle is inserted.

Common Thyroid Disease Complications

Thyroid Cancer Treatment

When a patient is confirmed as having thyroid cancer, via the tests that diagnose it, the treating doctor will refer the patient to a surgeon, who will determine how the cancer will need to be removed. If the cancer affects only one lobe of the thyroid (there are two lobes, one on each side), the surgeon may wish to perform what is called a "lobectomy", (partial thyroidectomy) meaning there will be removal of only one side of the gland.

If the surgeon feels removal of only one lobe, still places the patient at risk for the cancer returning, he may instead decide to remove the entire gland, which is referred to as a "total thyroidectomy". The type surgery is also determined by considering the type of thyroid cancer that is involved.

Some types of cancer are more aggressive than others and with these the surgeon will always recommend total thyroid removal. Surgeons also must determine at what stage the cancer is in, meaning how far it has progressed.

In order to decrease the risk of the cancer returning, the surgeon may also want to remove the lymph nodes in the neck, that are located near the thyroid gland. The lymph nodes may also be sent off for laboratory analysis to determine if they already contained cancer, which might then lead the surgeon to recommending further treatment.

Post Operative Thyroid Cancer Treatments

Additional treatment after any type of thyroidectomy might also include Radio Active Iodine Therapy (RAI) or Chemotherapy, to destroy any remaining thyroid tissue that is capable of absorbing iodine in the body or any remaining cancer cells.

Any remaining thyroid tissue that is capable of taking up iodine, which is what the thyroid mostly consists of, also has the ability to re-develop cancer cells and is the reason RAI is sometimes used following a Total Thyroidectomy. Chemotherapy is directed at any remaining cancer cells that might remain in the body after a Total Thyroidectomy.

Regardless of the type of thyroid surgery that is performed, thyroid hormone replacement therapy is always used following thyroid cancer surgeries. The goal of the hormone therapy is to suppress the patient's TSH level (pituitary hormone that decreases when thyroid hormone is increased). This also helps prevent recurrence of cancer but also replaces any hormone the thyroid gland is not capable of producing following surgery.

If a patient is given RAI after surgery, they may not be replaced with thyroid hormone for a month or two following the treatment. Most patients will need thyroid hormone replacement therapy following any type of thyroidectomy, as lifelong treatment.

The treatment for hypothyroidism following thyroid cancer is simply to "replace" the low hormone. This is done by giving the patient "thyroid hormone replacement medication". The Doctor will prescribe a starting dose for the patient and do follow-up blood testing to adjust the dose to the correct level over time, which is called "titrating" the dose.

Following are helpful suggestions for patients who are placed on thyroid hormone therapy following thyroid cancer treatment:

• Take your thyroid hormone medication on an empty stomach, with plenty of water.

• Take your thyroid hormone medication at the same time each day.

• If you take vitamins or supplements containing iron or calcium, be sure to take them six hours apart from your thyroid medication dose.

• When you have blood retests of your thyroid hormone levels, take your medication at the same time, to correlate with each blood draw.

• Never adjust your own thyroid medication dose.

Thyroid cancers have a very high treatment success rate but that success rate is even higher when thyroid cancers are diagnosed and treated early.

It is very important to see your doctor if you discover any nodules (tumor-like growths) on your thyroid gland or if you have difficulty swallowing or feel, that you might have a growth on the inside of your throat. This is also important if you experience the symptoms of either an overactive or under active thyroid gland.

CHAPTER FIFTEEN

Hashimoto's Encephalopathy Rare but Serious

There is a neuro-endocrine disorder that causes very serious and potentially life threatening symptoms, called Hashimoto's Encephalopathy (HE). The disorder can occur in patients with Hashimoto's thyroiditis, who experience a very high elevation of "thyroid antibody" levels. These antibodies, that attack the thyroid gland after recognition of it by the immune system, as a foreign invader, can become highly elevated in these rare cases of HE. At these high elevations they will begin to affect brain and nerve function in the body or the "neurological system". Severe symptoms will result because this system is the body's information and communication center and a disruption from a disease process can cause an array of nerve and brain related symptoms.

Inflammation caused by the antibodies (also called auto-antibodies) spreads to the brain and begins to affect the tissue containing the nerves that control bodily functions and impulses throughout the body.

The resulting effect, are severe neurological symptoms, meaning abnormal responses and manifestations of nervous system dysfunction. These symptoms can include; psychotic episodes (hallucinations and delusions, dementia (mental deterioration), neuropathies (abnormal nerve sensations) and even coma or death if left untreated.

The antibodies responsible for causing thyroid destruction and inflammation in the thyroid gland but that can also cause HE when highly elevated, are the "TPO" (anti-thyroidperoxidase) and "TG" (anti-thyroglobulin) antibodies. This autoimmune process, called Hashimoto's thyroiditis that can result in the less common Hashimoto's Encephalopathy, is more often a result of elevated anti-TPO levels although it can result from elevations of both it and the anti-TG antibodies.

Thyroid hormone levels are not usually a factor in this potentially serious neuro-endocrine disorder of thyroid autoimmunity. Some patients in fact have been documented in medical research, to have experienced HE with their thyroid hormone levels in normal range and before they were in need of thyroid hormone replacement therapy.

Common Thyroid Disease Complications

This disorder is a rare but a strong example of the fact that thyroid antibodies have the ability to produce bodily symptoms regardless of thyroid hormone levels.

Treatment for HE, is to reduce the inflammation caused by the thyroid antibodies by administering a steroid anti-inflammatory drug to patients who are diagnosed. These drugs, also called corticosteroids or hydrocortisone, mimic the anti-inflammatory properties of our body's own natural anti-inflammatory called "cortisol". A major brand prescribed for inflammatory conditions is "Prednisone", a powerful steroid that usually achieves an anti-inflammatory effect quickly with only a relatively short term regimen being necessary to correct cases of HE.

If a patient with Hashimoto's thyroiditis or their loved ones, notice the onset of sudden and severe neurological symptoms, they should report to their Doctor immediately, to rule out HE as the cause. A delay in treatment for a patient experiencing this very rare disorder could result in severe consequences.

It is my sincere hope that I have helped to provide a general understanding to the readers of this book, in regard to those complications that commonly, less-commonly and rarely occur with thyroid diseases and disorders.

(END)